100 Day Cystic Fibrosis Medical Log

Created by: Heidi Wildes Mitchell

Copyright 2018@Heidi Wildes Mitchell

All rights reserved

ISBN-13:
978-1726234184

ISBN-10:
1726234185

For my awesome son, Eli, I love you more than any words could ever describe. CF does not define you; it is just a small part of who you are!

Cystic Fibrosis Medical Log

Belongs to:

_____

_____

_____

_____

Note from the Author

For the users of this medical log,

I am not a medical doctor; I am the mom of a teenager with Cystic Fibrosis (CF). I created this log because I thought that it might come in handy for several different reasons. First, it can be overwhelming for new parents to this condition, so the log can help you manage the day-to-day regiment until you feel comfortable. Second, you may only want to use the log when a caregiver or babysitter is coming into your home. I know it's hard to remember everything and this can help you to keep it all organized. Third, it's also hard to remember the past couple of months when getting to your regularly scheduled CF clinic visits, so you may want to use it each day for reference during those visits. Finally, it can aide teenagers and adults with CF independently manage their condition. I've noticed my own child getting lax on some of the supplemental medications he takes and this log can help to minimize those occurrences.

I have included a chart with the most common medications taken by CF patients, but also added a few blank lines for any supplemental medications. On the back side of that page, you can keep track of diet recommendations, exercise (which is very important for increasing lung capacity), compression methods (for loosening any sputum in the lungs), and any additional information that may be helpful to yourself, caregivers or at doctor's appointments.

Whatever your purpose for using this medical log, I truly want it to be a positive tool in your arsenal for maintaining a healthy CF patient!

Heidi Wildes Mitchell

Emergency Contact Information

Pediatrician _____

Address _____

_____

CF Clinic _____

Address _____

_____

Endocrinologist _____

Address _____

_____

GI Specialist _____

Address _____

_____

Family Physician _____

Address _____

_____

School _____

Police Dept. _____

Fire Department _____

CDC _____

Upcoming Doctor Appointments:

Date: _____

Doctor: _____

Date & Time: _____

Doctor: _____

Date & Time: _____

Doctor: _____

Date & Time: _____

Doctor: _____

Date & Time: _____

Doctor: _____

Date & Time: _____

Doctor: _____

Date & Time: _____

Doctor: _____

Date: August 16, 2018 SAMPLE PAGE

Dispensed Medications:

Creon __36__ mg # with meals __5__ # with snacks __3__

	Dosage	Time
Breakfast	5 pills/enzymes	7 am
Snack	3 pills	10:30 am
Lunch	5 pills	1 pm
Snack	3 pills	4 pm
Dinner	5 pills	6:30 pm
Snack	N/A	

*Creon should always be given with a meal or snack, if it has been more than two hours since the last dosage. Do not administer generic brands of Creon.

Medication	Dosage	Times
Prevacid/Gas	1 times daily	7 am
Albuterol	2 times daily	6 am & 8 pm
Pulmozyme	1 times daily	8 pm
Saline	2 times daily	6 am & 8 pm
Multi-Vitamin	2 times daily	7 am & 6:30 pm
Specialty Vitamin	1 times weekly/4	7 am
Oral Antibiotic	N/A	
Inhale Antibiotic	N/A	
Nasal Spray	2 times daily	7 am & 7 pm
Miralax	N/A	
Cinnamon Pills	2 at one time	7 am

Daily Activity

Special dietary needs: SAMPLE PAGE

Three ensure drinks daily and use double cheese in Sandwich

_____

_____

_____

Exercise: Swim practice 4:30-5:30

	None	Light	Medium	Severe
Cough		x		
Sputum	x			

Stools # Daily ___2___   Greasy, Yes/NO   Color: Brown

Compression vest frequency: 2 times daily

Compression vest settings:

Intervals	Duration	Speed
1	10 minutes	10 HZ
2	10 min	12 HZ
3	10 min	15 HZ

Pep Device frequency: N/A

Additional Notes:

Vitamin D only given on Thursday

_____

_____

_____

_____

Date: _____

Dispensed Medications:

Creon _____ mg # with meals _____ # with snacks _____

	Dosage	Time
Breakfast		
Snack		
Lunch		
Snack		
Dinner		
Snack		

*Creon should always be given with a meal or snack, if it has been more than two hours since the last dosage. Do not administer generic brands of Creon.

Medication	Dosage	Times
Prevacid/Gas		
Albuterol		
Pulmozyme		
Saline		
Multi-Vitamin		
Specialty Vitamin		
Oral Antibiotic		
Inhale Antibiotic		
Nasal Spray		
Miralax		

Daily Activity

Special dietary needs:

_____
_____
_____
_____

Exercise: _____

	None	Light	Medium	Severe
Cough				
Sputum				

Stools # Daily _____ **Greasy, Yes/NO Color:** _____

Compression vest frequency: _____

Compression vest settings:

Intervals	Duration	Speed
1		
2		
3		

Pep Device frequency: _____

Additional Notes:

_____
_____
_____
_____
_____

Date: _____

Dispensed Medications:

Creon _____ mg # with meals _____ # with snacks _____

	Dosage	Time
Breakfast		
Snack		
Lunch		
Snack		
Dinner		
Snack		

*Creon should always be given with a meal or snack, if it has been more than two hours since the last dosage. Do not administer generic brands of Creon.

Medication	Dosage	Times
Prevacid/Gas		
Albuterol		
Pulmozyme		
Saline		
Multi-Vitamin		
Specialty Vitamin		
Oral Antibiotic		
Inhale Antibiotic		
Nasal Spray		
Miralax		

Daily Activity

Special dietary needs:

_____

_____

_____

_____

Exercise: _____

	None	Light	Medium	Severe
Cough				
Sputum				

Stools # Daily _____ **Greasy, Yes/NO Color:** _____

Compression vest frequency: _____

Compression vest settings:

Intervals	Duration	Speed
1		
2		
3		

Pep Device frequency: _____

Additional Notes:

_____

_____

_____

_____

_____

Date: _____

Dispensed Medications:

Creon _____ mg # with meals _____ # with snacks _____

	Dosage	Time
Breakfast		
Snack		
Lunch		
Snack		
Dinner		
Snack		

*Creon should always be given with a meal or snack, if it has been more than two hours since the last dosage. Do not administer generic brands of Creon.

Medication	Dosage	Times
Prevacid/Gas		
Albuterol		
Pulmozyme		
Saline		
Multi-Vitamin		
Specialty Vitamin		
Oral Antibiotic		
Inhale Antibiotic		
Nasal Spray		
Miralax		

Daily Activity

Special dietary needs:

_____

_____

_____

_____

Exercise: _____

	None	Light	Medium	Severe
Cough				
Sputum				

Stools # Daily _____ **Greasy, Yes/NO Color:** _____

Compression vest frequency: _____

Compression vest settings:

Intervals	Duration	Speed
1		
2		
3		

Pep Device frequency: _____

Additional Notes:

_____

_____

_____

_____

_____

Date: _____

Dispensed Medications:

Creon _____ mg # with meals _____ # with snacks_____

	Dosage	Time
Breakfast		
Snack		
Lunch		
Snack		
Dinner		
Snack		

*Creon should always be given with a meal or snack, if it has been more than two hours since the last dosage. Do not administer generic brands of Creon.

Medication	Dosage	Times
Prevacid/Gas		
Albuterol		
Pulmozyme		
Saline		
Multi-Vitamin		
Specialty Vitamin		
Oral Antibiotic		
Inhale Antibiotic		
Nasal Spray		
Miralax		

Daily Activity

Special dietary needs:

_____

_____

_____

_____

Exercise: _____

	None	Light	Medium	Severe
Cough				
Sputum				

Stools # Daily _____ **Greasy, Yes/NO Color:** _____

Compression vest frequency: _____

Compression vest settings:

Intervals	Duration	Speed
1		
2		
3		

Pep Device frequency: _____

Additional Notes:

_____

_____

_____

_____

Date: _____

Dispensed Medications:

Creon _____mg # with meals _____ # with snacks_____

	Dosage	Time
Breakfast		
Snack		
Lunch		
Snack		
Dinner		
Snack		

*Creon should always be given with a meal or snack, if it has been more than two hours since the last dosage. Do not administer generic brands of Creon.

Medication	Dosage	Times
Prevacid/Gas		
Albuterol		
Pulmozyme		
Saline		
Multi-Vitamin		
Specialty Vitamin		
Oral Antibiotic		
Inhale Antibiotic		
Nasal Spray		
Miralax		

Daily Activity

Special dietary needs:

_____

_____

_____

_____

Exercise: _____

	None	Light	Medium	Severe
Cough				
Sputum				

Stools # Daily _____ **Greasy, Yes/NO Color:** _____

Compression vest frequency: _____

Compression vest settings:

Intervals	Duration	Speed
1		
2		
3		

Pep Device frequency: _____

Additional Notes:

_____

_____

_____

_____

Date: _____

Dispensed Medications:

Creon _____ mg # with meals _____ # with snacks _____

	Dosage	Time
Breakfast		
Snack		
Lunch		
Snack		
Dinner		
Snack		

*Creon should always be given with a meal or snack, if it has been more than two hours since the last dosage. Do not administer generic brands of Creon.

Medication	Dosage	Times
Prevacid/Gas		
Albuterol		
Pulmozyme		
Saline		
Multi-Vitamin		
Specialty Vitamin		
Oral Antibiotic		
Inhale Antibiotic		
Nasal Spray		
Miralax		

Daily Activity

Special dietary needs:

_____

_____

_____

_____

Exercise: _____

	None	Light	Medium	Severe
Cough				
Sputum				

Stools # Daily _____ **Greasy, Yes/NO Color:** _____

Compression vest frequency: _____

Compression vest settings:

Intervals	Duration	Speed
1		
2		
3		

Pep Device frequency: _____

Additional Notes:

_____

_____

_____

_____

_____

Date: _____

Dispensed Medications:

Creon _____mg # with meals _____ # with snacks_____

	Dosage	Time
Breakfast		
Snack		
Lunch		
Snack		
Dinner		
Snack		

*Creon should always be given with a meal or snack, if it has been more than two hours since the last dosage. Do not administer generic brands of Creon.

Medication	Dosage	Times
Prevacid/Gas		
Albuterol		
Pulmozyme		
Saline		
Multi-Vitamin		
Specialty Vitamin		
Oral Antibiotic		
Inhale Antibiotic		
Nasal Spray		
Miralax		

Daily Activity

Special dietary needs:

_____

_____

_____

_____

Exercise: _____

	None	Light	Medium	Severe
Cough				
Sputum				

Stools # Daily _____ **Greasy, Yes/NO Color:** _____

Compression vest frequency: _____

Compression vest settings:

Intervals	Duration	Speed
1		
2		
3		

Pep Device frequency: _____

Additional Notes:

_____

_____

_____

_____

_____

Date: _____

Dispensed Medications:

Creon _____ mg # with meals _____ # with snacks _____

	Dosage	Time
Breakfast		
Snack		
Lunch		
Snack		
Dinner		
Snack		

*Creon should always be given with a meal or snack, if it has been more than two hours since the last dosage. Do not administer generic brands of Creon.

Medication	Dosage	Times
Prevacid/Gas		
Albuterol		
Pulmozyme		
Saline		
Multi-Vitamin		
Specialty Vitamin		
Oral Antibiotic		
Inhale Antibiotic		
Nasal Spray		
Miralax		

Daily Activity

Special dietary needs:

_____
_____
_____
_____

Exercise: _____

	None	Light	Medium	Severe
Cough				
Sputum				

Stools # Daily _____ **Greasy, Yes/NO Color:** _____

Compression vest frequency: _____

Compression vest settings:

Intervals	Duration	Speed
1		
2		
3		

Pep Device frequency: _____

Additional Notes:

_____
_____
_____
_____
_____

Date: _____

Dispensed Medications:

Creon _____mg # with meals _____ # with snacks_____

	Dosage	Time
Breakfast		
Snack		
Lunch		
Snack		
Dinner		
Snack		

*Creon should always be given with a meal or snack, if it has been more than two hours since the last dosage. Do not administer generic brands of Creon.

Medication	Dosage	Times
Prevacid/Gas		
Albuterol		
Pulmozyme		
Saline		
Multi-Vitamin		
Specialty Vitamin		
Oral Antibiotic		
Inhale Antibiotic		
Nasal Spray		
Miralax		

Daily Activity

Special dietary needs:

_____

_____

_____

_____

Exercise: _____

	None	Light	Medium	Severe
Cough				
Sputum				

Stools # Daily _____ **Greasy, Yes/NO Color:** _____

Compression vest frequency: _____

Compression vest settings:

Intervals	Duration	Speed
1		
2		
3		

Pep Device frequency: _____

Additional Notes:

_____

_____

_____

_____

Date: _____

Dispensed Medications:

Creon _____mg # with meals _____ # with snacks_____

	Dosage	Time
Breakfast		
Snack		
Lunch		
Snack		
Dinner		
Snack		

*Creon should always be given with a meal or snack, if it has been more than two hours since the last dosage. Do not administer generic brands of Creon.

Medication	Dosage	Times
Prevacid/Gas		
Albuterol		
Pulmozyme		
Saline		
Multi-Vitamin		
Specialty Vitamin		
Oral Antibiotic		
Inhale Antibiotic		
Nasal Spray		
Miralax		

Daily Activity

Special dietary needs:

_____

_____

_____

_____

Exercise: _____

	None	Light	Medium	Severe
Cough				
Sputum				

Stools # Daily _____ **Greasy, Yes/NO Color:** _____

Compression vest frequency: _____

Compression vest settings:

Intervals	Duration	Speed
1		
2		
3		

Pep Device frequency: _____

Additional Notes:

_____

_____

_____

_____

_____

Date: _____

Dispensed Medications:

Creon _____ mg # with meals _____ # with snacks _____

	Dosage	Time
Breakfast		
Snack		
Lunch		
Snack		
Dinner		
Snack		

*Creon should always be given with a meal or snack, if it has been more than two hours since the last dosage. Do not administer generic brands of Creon.

Medication	Dosage	Times
Prevacid/Gas		
Albuterol		
Pulmozyme		
Saline		
Multi-Vitamin		
Specialty Vitamin		
Oral Antibiotic		
Inhale Antibiotic		
Nasal Spray		
Miralax		

Daily Activity

Special dietary needs:

_____

_____

_____

_____

Exercise: _____

	None	Light	Medium	Severe
Cough				
Sputum				

Stools # Daily _____ **Greasy, Yes/NO Color:** _____

Compression vest frequency: _____

Compression vest settings:

Intervals	Duration	Speed
1		
2		
3		

Pep Device frequency: _____

Additional Notes:

_____

_____

_____

_____

Date: _____

Dispensed Medications:

Creon _____ mg # with meals _____ # with snacks _____

	Dosage	Time
Breakfast		
Snack		
Lunch		
Snack		
Dinner		
Snack		

*Creon should always be given with a meal or snack, if it has been more than two hours since the last dosage. Do not administer generic brands of Creon.

Medication	Dosage	Times
Prevacid/Gas		
Albuterol		
Pulmozyme		
Saline		
Multi-Vitamin		
Specialty Vitamin		
Oral Antibiotic		
Inhale Antibiotic		
Nasal Spray		
Miralax		

Daily Activity

Special dietary needs:

_____

_____

_____

_____

Exercise: _____

	None	Light	Medium	Severe
Cough				
Sputum				

Stools # Daily _____ **Greasy, Yes/NO Color:** _____

Compression vest frequency: _____

Compression vest settings:

Intervals	Duration	Speed
1		
2		
3		

Pep Device frequency: _____

Additional Notes:

_____

_____

_____

_____

_____

Date: _____

Dispensed Medications:

Creon _____ mg # with meals _____ # with snacks _____

	Dosage	Time
Breakfast		
Snack		
Lunch		
Snack		
Dinner		
Snack		

*Creon should always be given with a meal or snack, if it has been more than two hours since the last dosage. Do not administer generic brands of Creon.

Medication	Dosage	Times
Prevacid/Gas		
Albuterol		
Pulmozyme		
Saline		
Multi-Vitamin		
Specialty Vitamin		
Oral Antibiotic		
Inhale Antibiotic		
Nasal Spray		
Miralax		

Daily Activity

Special dietary needs:

_____

_____

_____

_____

Exercise: _____

	None	Light	Medium	Severe
Cough				
Sputum				

Stools # Daily _____ **Greasy, Yes/NO Color:** _____

Compression vest frequency: _____

Compression vest settings:

Intervals	Duration	Speed
1		
2		
3		

Pep Device frequency: _____

Additional Notes:

_____

_____

_____

_____

_____

Date: _____

Dispensed Medications:

Creon _____ mg # with meals _____ # with snacks _____

	Dosage	Time
Breakfast		
Snack		
Lunch		
Snack		
Dinner		
Snack		

*Creon should always be given with a meal or snack, if it has been more than two hours since the last dosage. Do not administer generic brands of Creon.

Medication	Dosage	Times
Prevacid/Gas		
Albuterol		
Pulmozyme		
Saline		
Multi-Vitamin		
Specialty Vitamin		
Oral Antibiotic		
Inhale Antibiotic		
Nasal Spray		
Miralax		

Daily Activity

Special dietary needs:
_____
_____
_____
_____

Exercise: _____

	None	Light	Medium	Severe
Cough				
Sputum				

Stools # Daily _____ **Greasy, Yes/NO Color:** _____

Compression vest frequency: _____

Compression vest settings:

Intervals	Duration	Speed
1		
2		
3		

Pep Device frequency: _____

Additional Notes:
_____
_____
_____
_____
_____

Date: _____

Dispensed Medications:

Creon _____ mg # with meals _____ # with snacks _____

	Dosage	Time
Breakfast		
Snack		
Lunch		
Snack		
Dinner		
Snack		

*Creon should always be given with a meal or snack, if it has been more than two hours since the last dosage. Do not administer generic brands of Creon.

Medication	Dosage	Times
Prevacid/Gas		
Albuterol		
Pulmozyme		
Saline		
Multi-Vitamin		
Specialty Vitamin		
Oral Antibiotic		
Inhale Antibiotic		
Nasal Spray		
Miralax		

Daily Activity

Special dietary needs:

_____

_____

_____

_____

Exercise: _____

	None	Light	Medium	Severe
Cough				
Sputum				

Stools # Daily _____ **Greasy, Yes/NO Color:** _____

Compression vest frequency: _____

Compression vest settings:

Intervals	Duration	Speed
1		
2		
3		

Pep Device frequency: _____

Additional Notes:

_____

_____

_____

_____

_____

Date: _____

Dispensed Medications:

Creon _____mg # with meals _____ # with snacks_____

	Dosage	Time
Breakfast		
Snack		
Lunch		
Snack		
Dinner		
Snack		

*Creon should always be given with a meal or snack, if it has been more than two hours since the last dosage. Do not administer generic brands of Creon.

Medication	Dosage	Times
Prevacid/Gas		
Albuterol		
Pulmozyme		
Saline		
Multi-Vitamin		
Specialty Vitamin		
Oral Antibiotic		
Inhale Antibiotic		
Nasal Spray		
Miralax		

Daily Activity

Special dietary needs:

_____

_____

_____

_____

Exercise: _____

	None	Light	Medium	Severe
Cough				
Sputum				

Stools # Daily _____ **Greasy, Yes/NO Color:** _____

Compression vest frequency: _____

Compression vest settings:

Intervals	Duration	Speed
1		
2		
3		

Pep Device frequency: _____

Additional Notes:

_____

_____

_____

_____

_____

Date: _____

Dispensed Medications:

Creon _____mg # with meals _____ # with snacks_____

	Dosage	Time
Breakfast		
Snack		
Lunch		
Snack		
Dinner		
Snack		

*Creon should always be given with a meal or snack, if it has been more than two hours since the last dosage. Do not administer generic brands of Creon.

Medication	Dosage	Times
Prevacid/Gas		
Albuterol		
Pulmozyme		
Saline		
Multi-Vitamin		
Specialty Vitamin		
Oral Antibiotic		
Inhale Antibiotic		
Nasal Spray		
Miralax		

Daily Activity

Special dietary needs:

_____
_____
_____
_____

Exercise: _____

	None	Light	Medium	Severe
Cough				
Sputum				

Stools # Daily _____ **Greasy, Yes/NO Color:** _____

Compression vest frequency: _____

Compression vest settings:

Intervals	Duration	Speed
1		
2		
3		

Pep Device frequency: _____

Additional Notes:

_____
_____
_____
_____
_____

Date: _____

Dispensed Medications:

Creon _____ mg # with meals _____ # with snacks _____

	Dosage	Time
Breakfast		
Snack		
Lunch		
Snack		
Dinner		
Snack		

*Creon should always be given with a meal or snack, if it has been more than two hours since the last dosage. Do not administer generic brands of Creon.

Medication	Dosage	Times
Prevacid/Gas		
Albuterol		
Pulmozyme		
Saline		
Multi-Vitamin		
Specialty Vitamin		
Oral Antibiotic		
Inhale Antibiotic		
Nasal Spray		
Miralax		

Daily Activity

Special dietary needs:

_____

_____

_____

_____

Exercise: _____

	None	Light	Medium	Severe
Cough				
Sputum				

Stools # Daily _____ **Greasy, Yes/NO Color:** _____

Compression vest frequency: _____

Compression vest settings:

Intervals	Duration	Speed
1		
2		
3		

Pep Device frequency: _____

Additional Notes:

_____

_____

_____

_____

_____

Date: _____

Dispensed Medications:

Creon _____mg # with meals _____ # with snacks_____

	Dosage	Time
Breakfast		
Snack		
Lunch		
Snack		
Dinner		
Snack		

*Creon should always be given with a meal or snack, if it has been more than two hours since the last dosage. Do not administer generic brands of Creon.

Medication	Dosage	Times
Prevacid/Gas		
Albuterol		
Pulmozyme		
Saline		
Multi-Vitamin		
Specialty Vitamin		
Oral Antibiotic		
Inhale Antibiotic		
Nasal Spray		
Miralax		

Daily Activity

Special dietary needs:

_____

_____

_____

_____

Exercise: _____

	None	Light	Medium	Severe
Cough				
Sputum				

Stools # Daily _____ **Greasy, Yes/NO Color:** _____

Compression vest frequency: _____

Compression vest settings:

Intervals	Duration	Speed
1		
2		
3		

Pep Device frequency: _____

Additional Notes:

_____

_____

_____

_____

_____

Date: _____

Dispensed Medications:

Creon _____ mg # with meals _____ # with snacks_____

	Dosage	Time
Breakfast		
Snack		
Lunch		
Snack		
Dinner		
Snack		

*Creon should always be given with a meal or snack, if it has been more than two hours since the last dosage. Do not administer generic brands of Creon.

Medication	Dosage	Times
Prevacid/Gas		
Albuterol		
Pulmozyme		
Saline		
Multi-Vitamin		
Specialty Vitamin		
Oral Antibiotic		
Inhale Antibiotic		
Nasal Spray		
Miralax		

Daily Activity

Special dietary needs:

_____
_____
_____
_____

Exercise: _____

	None	Light	Medium	Severe
Cough				
Sputum				

Stools # Daily _____ **Greasy, Yes/NO Color:** _____

Compression vest frequency: _____

Compression vest settings:

Intervals	Duration	Speed
1		
2		
3		

Pep Device frequency: _____

Additional Notes:

_____
_____
_____
_____
_____

Date: _____

Dispensed Medications:

Creon _____ mg # with meals _____ # with snacks _____

	Dosage	Time
Breakfast		
Snack		
Lunch		
Snack		
Dinner		
Snack		

*Creon should always be given with a meal or snack, if it has been more than two hours since the last dosage. Do not administer generic brands of Creon.

Medication	Dosage	Times
Prevacid/Gas		
Albuterol		
Pulmozyme		
Saline		
Multi-Vitamin		
Specialty Vitamin		
Oral Antibiotic		
Inhale Antibiotic		
Nasal Spray		
Miralax		

Daily Activity

Special dietary needs:

_____

_____

_____

_____

Exercise: _____

	None	Light	Medium	Severe
Cough				
Sputum				

Stools # Daily _____ **Greasy, Yes/NO Color:** _____

Compression vest frequency: _____

Compression vest settings:

Intervals	Duration	Speed
1		
2		
3		

Pep Device frequency: _____

Additional Notes:

_____

_____

_____

_____

_____

Date: _____

Dispensed Medications:

Creon _____mg # with meals _____ # with snacks_____

	Dosage	Time
Breakfast		
Snack		
Lunch		
Snack		
Dinner		
Snack		

*Creon should always be given with a meal or snack, if it has been more than two hours since the last dosage. Do not administer generic brands of Creon.

Medication	Dosage	Times
Prevacid/Gas		
Albuterol		
Pulmozyme		
Saline		
Multi-Vitamin		
Specialty Vitamin		
Oral Antibiotic		
Inhale Antibiotic		
Nasal Spray		
Miralax		

Daily Activity

Special dietary needs:

_____

_____

_____

_____

Exercise: _____

	None	Light	Medium	Severe
Cough				
Sputum				

Stools # Daily _____ **Greasy, Yes/NO Color:** _____

Compression vest frequency: _____

Compression vest settings:

Intervals	Duration	Speed
1		
2		
3		

Pep Device frequency: _____

Additional Notes:

_____

_____

_____

_____

Date: _____

Dispensed Medications:

Creon _____ mg # with meals _____ # with snacks _____

	Dosage	Time
Breakfast		
Snack		
Lunch		
Snack		
Dinner		
Snack		

*Creon should always be given with a meal or snack, if it has been more than two hours since the last dosage. Do not administer generic brands of Creon.

Medication	Dosage	Times
Prevacid/Gas		
Albuterol		
Pulmozyme		
Saline		
Multi-Vitamin		
Specialty Vitamin		
Oral Antibiotic		
Inhale Antibiotic		
Nasal Spray		
Miralax		

Daily Activity

Special dietary needs:

_____

_____

_____

_____

Exercise: _____

	None	Light	Medium	Severe
Cough				
Sputum				

Stools # Daily _____ **Greasy, Yes/NO Color:** _____

Compression vest frequency: _____

Compression vest settings:

Intervals	Duration	Speed
1		
2		
3		

Pep Device frequency: _____

Additional Notes:

_____

_____

_____

_____

_____

Date: _____

Dispensed Medications:

Creon _____ mg # with meals _____ # with snacks _____

	Dosage	Time
Breakfast		
Snack		
Lunch		
Snack		
Dinner		
Snack		

*Creon should always be given with a meal or snack, if it has been more than two hours since the last dosage. Do not administer generic brands of Creon.

Medication	Dosage	Times
Prevacid/Gas		
Albuterol		
Pulmozyme		
Saline		
Multi-Vitamin		
Specialty Vitamin		
Oral Antibiotic		
Inhale Antibiotic		
Nasal Spray		
Miralax		

Daily Activity

Special dietary needs:

_____

_____

_____

_____

Exercise: _____

	None	Light	Medium	Severe
Cough				
Sputum				

Stools # Daily _____ **Greasy, Yes/NO Color:** _____

Compression vest frequency: _____

Compression vest settings:

Intervals	Duration	Speed
1		
2		
3		

Pep Device frequency: _____

Additional Notes:

_____

_____

_____

_____

Date: _____

Dispensed Medications:

Creon _____mg # with meals _____ # with snacks_____

	Dosage	Time
Breakfast		
Snack		
Lunch		
Snack		
Dinner		
Snack		

*Creon should always be given with a meal or snack, if it has been more than two hours since the last dosage. Do not administer generic brands of Creon.

Medication	Dosage	Times
Prevacid/Gas		
Albuterol		
Pulmozyme		
Saline		
Multi-Vitamin		
Specialty Vitamin		
Oral Antibiotic		
Inhale Antibiotic		
Nasal Spray		
Miralax		

Daily Activity

Special dietary needs:

_____

_____

_____

_____

Exercise: _____

	None	Light	Medium	Severe
Cough				
Sputum				

Stools # Daily _____ **Greasy, Yes/NO Color:** _____

Compression vest frequency: _____

Compression vest settings:

Intervals	Duration	Speed
1		
2		
3		

Pep Device frequency: _____

Additional Notes:

_____

_____

_____

_____

Date: _____

Dispensed Medications:

Creon _____mg # with meals _____ # with snacks_____

	Dosage	Time
Breakfast		
Snack		
Lunch		
Snack		
Dinner		
Snack		

*Creon should always be given with a meal or snack, if it has been more than two hours since the last dosage. Do not administer generic brands of Creon.

Medication	Dosage	Times
Prevacid/Gas		
Albuterol		
Pulmozyme		
Saline		
Multi-Vitamin		
Specialty Vitamin		
Oral Antibiotic		
Inhale Antibiotic		
Nasal Spray		
Miralax		

Daily Activity

Special dietary needs:

_____

_____

_____

_____

Exercise: _____

	None	Light	Medium	Severe
Cough				
Sputum				

Stools # Daily _____ **Greasy, Yes/NO Color:** _____

Compression vest frequency: _____

Compression vest settings:

Intervals	Duration	Speed
1		
2		
3		

Pep Device frequency: _____

Additional Notes:

_____

_____

_____

_____

_____

Date: _____

Dispensed Medications:

Creon _____ mg # with meals _____ # with snacks _____

	Dosage	Time
Breakfast		
Snack		
Lunch		
Snack		
Dinner		
Snack		

*Creon should always be given with a meal or snack, if it has been more than two hours since the last dosage. Do not administer generic brands of Creon.

Medication	Dosage	Times
Prevacid/Gas		
Albuterol		
Pulmozyme		
Saline		
Multi-Vitamin		
Specialty Vitamin		
Oral Antibiotic		
Inhale Antibiotic		
Nasal Spray		
Miralax		

Daily Activity

Special dietary needs:

_____

_____

_____

_____

Exercise: _____

	None	Light	Medium	Severe
Cough				
Sputum				

Stools # Daily _____ **Greasy, Yes/NO Color:** _____

Compression vest frequency: _____

Compression vest settings:

Intervals	Duration	Speed
1		
2		
3		

Pep Device frequency: _____

Additional Notes:

_____

_____

_____

_____

_____

Date: _____

Dispensed Medications:

Creon _____mg # with meals _____ # with snacks_____

	Dosage	Time
Breakfast		
Snack		
Lunch		
Snack		
Dinner		
Snack		

*Creon should always be given with a meal or snack, if it has been more than two hours since the last dosage. Do not administer generic brands of Creon.

Medication	Dosage	Times
Prevacid/Gas		
Albuterol		
Pulmozyme		
Saline		
Multi-Vitamin		
Specialty Vitamin		
Oral Antibiotic		
Inhale Antibiotic		
Nasal Spray		
Miralax		

Daily Activity

Special dietary needs:

_____

_____

_____

_____

Exercise: _____

	None	Light	Medium	Severe
Cough				
Sputum				

Stools # Daily _____ **Greasy, Yes/NO Color:** _____

Compression vest frequency: _____

Compression vest settings:

Intervals	Duration	Speed
1		
2		
3		

Pep Device frequency: _____

Additional Notes:

_____

_____

_____

_____

_____

Date: _____

Dispensed Medications:

Creon _____mg # with meals _____ # with snacks_____

	Dosage	Time
Breakfast		
Snack		
Lunch		
Snack		
Dinner		
Snack		

*Creon should always be given with a meal or snack, if it has been more than two hours since the last dosage. Do not administer generic brands of Creon.

Medication	Dosage	Times
Prevacid/Gas		
Albuterol		
Pulmozyme		
Saline		
Multi-Vitamin		
Specialty Vitamin		
Oral Antibiotic		
Inhale Antibiotic		
Nasal Spray		
Miralax		

Daily Activity

Special dietary needs:

_____

_____

_____

_____

Exercise: _____

	None	Light	Medium	Severe
Cough				
Sputum				

Stools # Daily _____ **Greasy, Yes/NO Color:** _____

Compression vest frequency: _____

Compression vest settings:

Intervals	Duration	Speed
1		
2		
3		

Pep Device frequency: _____

Additional Notes:

_____

_____

_____

_____

_____

Date: _____

Dispensed Medications:

Creon _____mg # with meals _____ # with snacks_____

	Dosage	Time
Breakfast		
Snack		
Lunch		
Snack		
Dinner		
Snack		

*Creon should always be given with a meal or snack, if it has been more than two hours since the last dosage. Do not administer generic brands of Creon.

Medication	Dosage	Times
Prevacid/Gas		
Albuterol		
Pulmozyme		
Saline		
Multi-Vitamin		
Specialty Vitamin		
Oral Antibiotic		
Inhale Antibiotic		
Nasal Spray		
Miralax		

Daily Activity

Special dietary needs:

_____

_____

_____

_____

Exercise: _____

	None	Light	Medium	Severe
Cough				
Sputum				

Stools # Daily _____ **Greasy, Yes/NO Color:** _____

Compression vest frequency: _____

Compression vest settings:

Intervals	Duration	Speed
1		
2		
3		

Pep Device frequency: _____

Additional Notes:

_____

_____

_____

_____

_____

Date: _____

Dispensed Medications:

Creon _____mg # with meals _____ # with snacks_____

	Dosage	Time
Breakfast		
Snack		
Lunch		
Snack		
Dinner		
Snack		

*Creon should always be given with a meal or snack, if it has been more than two hours since the last dosage. Do not administer generic brands of Creon.

Medication	Dosage	Times
Prevacid/Gas		
Albuterol		
Pulmozyme		
Saline		
Multi-Vitamin		
Specialty Vitamin		
Oral Antibiotic		
Inhale Antibiotic		
Nasal Spray		
Miralax		

Daily Activity

Special dietary needs:
_____
_____
_____
_____

Exercise: _____

	None	Light	Medium	Severe
Cough				
Sputum				

Stools # Daily _____ **Greasy, Yes/NO Color:** _____

Compression vest frequency: _____

Compression vest settings:

Intervals	Duration	Speed
1		
2		
3		

Pep Device frequency: _____

Additional Notes:
_____
_____
_____
_____
_____

Date: _____

Dispensed Medications:

Creon _____mg # with meals _____ # with snacks_____

	Dosage	Time
Breakfast		
Snack		
Lunch		
Snack		
Dinner		
Snack		

*Creon should always be given with a meal or snack, if it has been more than two hours since the last dosage. Do not administer generic brands of Creon.

Medication	Dosage	Times
Prevacid/Gas		
Albuterol		
Pulmozyme		
Saline		
Multi-Vitamin		
Specialty Vitamin		
Oral Antibiotic		
Inhale Antibiotic		
Nasal Spray		
Miralax		

Daily Activity

Special dietary needs:

_____
_____
_____
_____

Exercise: _____

	None	Light	Medium	Severe
Cough				
Sputum				

Stools # Daily _____ **Greasy, Yes/NO Color:** _____

Compression vest frequency: _____

Compression vest settings:

Intervals	Duration	Speed
1		
2		
3		

Pep Device frequency: _____

Additional Notes:

_____
_____
_____
_____
_____

Date: _____

Dispensed Medications:

Creon _____ mg # with meals _____ # with snacks _____

	Dosage	Time
Breakfast		
Snack		
Lunch		
Snack		
Dinner		
Snack		

*Creon should always be given with a meal or snack, if it has been more than two hours since the last dosage. Do not administer generic brands of Creon.

Medication	Dosage	Times
Prevacid/Gas		
Albuterol		
Pulmozyme		
Saline		
Multi-Vitamin		
Specialty Vitamin		
Oral Antibiotic		
Inhale Antibiotic		
Nasal Spray		
Miralax		

Daily Activity

Special dietary needs:

_____

_____

_____

_____

Exercise: _____

	None	Light	Medium	Severe
Cough				
Sputum				

Stools # Daily _____ **Greasy, Yes/NO Color:** _____

Compression vest frequency: _____

Compression vest settings:

Intervals	Duration	Speed
1		
2		
3		

Pep Device frequency: _____

Additional Notes:

_____

_____

_____

_____

_____

Date: _____

Dispensed Medications:

Creon _____mg # with meals _____ # with snacks_____

	Dosage	Time
Breakfast		
Snack		
Lunch		
Snack		
Dinner		
Snack		

*Creon should always be given with a meal or snack, if it has been more than two hours since the last dosage. Do not administer generic brands of Creon.

Medication	Dosage	Times
Prevacid/Gas		
Albuterol		
Pulmozyme		
Saline		
Multi-Vitamin		
Specialty Vitamin		
Oral Antibiotic		
Inhale Antibiotic		
Nasal Spray		
Miralax		

Daily Activity

Special dietary needs:

_____

_____

_____

_____

Exercise: _____

	None	Light	Medium	Severe
Cough				
Sputum				

Stools # Daily _____ **Greasy, Yes/NO Color:** _____

Compression vest frequency: _____

Compression vest settings:

Intervals	Duration	Speed
1		
2		
3		

Pep Device frequency: _____

Additional Notes:

_____

_____

_____

_____

_____

Date: _____

Dispensed Medications:

Creon _____mg # with meals _____ # with snacks_____

	Dosage	Time
Breakfast		
Snack		
Lunch		
Snack		
Dinner		
Snack		

*Creon should always be given with a meal or snack, if it has been more than two hours since the last dosage. Do not administer generic brands of Creon.

Medication	Dosage	Times
Prevacid/Gas		
Albuterol		
Pulmozyme		
Saline		
Multi-Vitamin		
Specialty Vitamin		
Oral Antibiotic		
Inhale Antibiotic		
Nasal Spray		
Miralax		

Daily Activity

Special dietary needs:

_____

_____

_____

_____

Exercise: _____

	None	Light	Medium	Severe
Cough				
Sputum				

Stools # Daily _____ **Greasy, Yes/NO Color:** _____

Compression vest frequency: _____

Compression vest settings:

Intervals	Duration	Speed
1		
2		
3		

Pep Device frequency: _____

Additional Notes:

_____

_____

_____

_____

_____

Date: _____

Dispensed Medications:

Creon _____ mg # with meals _____ # with snacks _____

	Dosage	Time
Breakfast		
Snack		
Lunch		
Snack		
Dinner		
Snack		

*Creon should always be given with a meal or snack, if it has been more than two hours since the last dosage. Do not administer generic brands of Creon.

Medication	Dosage	Times
Prevacid/Gas		
Albuterol		
Pulmozyme		
Saline		
Multi-Vitamin		
Specialty Vitamin		
Oral Antibiotic		
Inhale Antibiotic		
Nasal Spray		
Miralax		

Daily Activity

Special dietary needs:

_____

_____

_____

_____

Exercise: _____

	None	Light	Medium	Severe
Cough				
Sputum				

Stools # Daily _____ **Greasy, Yes/NO Color:** _____

Compression vest frequency: _____

Compression vest settings:

Intervals	Duration	Speed
1		
2		
3		

Pep Device frequency: _____

Additional Notes:

_____

_____

_____

_____

_____

Date: _____

Dispensed Medications:

Creon _____mg # with meals _____ # with snacks_____

	Dosage	Time
Breakfast		
Snack		
Lunch		
Snack		
Dinner		
Snack		

*Creon should always be given with a meal or snack, if it has been more than two hours since the last dosage. Do not administer generic brands of Creon.

Medication	Dosage	Times
Prevacid/Gas		
Albuterol		
Pulmozyme		
Saline		
Multi-Vitamin		
Specialty Vitamin		
Oral Antibiotic		
Inhale Antibiotic		
Nasal Spray		
Miralax		

Daily Activity

Special dietary needs:

_____

_____

_____

_____

Exercise: _____

	None	Light	Medium	Severe
Cough				
Sputum				

Stools # Daily _____ **Greasy, Yes/NO Color:** _____

Compression vest frequency: _____

Compression vest settings:

Intervals	Duration	Speed
1		
2		
3		

Pep Device frequency: _____

Additional Notes:

_____

_____

_____

_____

_____

Date: _____

Dispensed Medications:

Creon _____mg # with meals _____ # with snacks_____

	Dosage	Time
Breakfast		
Snack		
Lunch		
Snack		
Dinner		
Snack		

*Creon should always be given with a meal or snack, if it has been more than two hours since the last dosage. Do not administer generic brands of Creon.

Medication	Dosage	Times
Prevacid/Gas		
Albuterol		
Pulmozyme		
Saline		
Multi-Vitamin		
Specialty Vitamin		
Oral Antibiotic		
Inhale Antibiotic		
Nasal Spray		
Miralax		

Daily Activity

Special dietary needs:

_____
_____
_____
_____

Exercise: _____

	None	Light	Medium	Severe
Cough				
Sputum				

Stools # Daily _____ **Greasy, Yes/NO Color:** _____

Compression vest frequency: _____

Compression vest settings:

Intervals	Duration	Speed
1		
2		
3		

Pep Device frequency: _____

Additional Notes:

_____
_____
_____
_____
_____

Date: _____

Dispensed Medications:

Creon _____mg # with meals _____ # with snacks_____

	Dosage	Time
Breakfast		
Snack		
Lunch		
Snack		
Dinner		
Snack		

*Creon should always be given with a meal or snack, if it has been more than two hours since the last dosage. Do not administer generic brands of Creon.

Medication	Dosage	Times
Prevacid/Gas		
Albuterol		
Pulmozyme		
Saline		
Multi-Vitamin		
Specialty Vitamin		
Oral Antibiotic		
Inhale Antibiotic		
Nasal Spray		
Miralax		

Daily Activity

Special dietary needs:

_____

_____

_____

_____

Exercise: _____

	None	Light	Medium	Severe
Cough				
Sputum				

Stools # Daily _____ **Greasy, Yes/NO Color:** _____

Compression vest frequency: _____

Compression vest settings:

Intervals	Duration	Speed
1		
2		
3		

Pep Device frequency: _____

Additional Notes:

_____

_____

_____

_____

Date: _____

Dispensed Medications:

Creon _____ mg # with meals _____ # with snacks _____

	Dosage	Time
Breakfast		
Snack		
Lunch		
Snack		
Dinner		
Snack		

*Creon should always be given with a meal or snack, if it has been more than two hours since the last dosage. Do not administer generic brands of Creon.

Medication	Dosage	Times
Prevacid/Gas		
Albuterol		
Pulmozyme		
Saline		
Multi-Vitamin		
Specialty Vitamin		
Oral Antibiotic		
Inhale Antibiotic		
Nasal Spray		
Miralax		

Daily Activity

Special dietary needs:

_____

_____

_____

_____

Exercise: _____

	None	Light	Medium	Severe
Cough				
Sputum				

Stools # Daily _____ **Greasy, Yes/NO Color:** _____

Compression vest frequency: _____

Compression vest settings:

Intervals	Duration	Speed
1		
2		
3		

Pep Device frequency: _____

Additional Notes:

_____

_____

_____

_____

Date: _____

Dispensed Medications:

Creon _____mg # with meals _____ # with snacks_____

	Dosage	Time
Breakfast		
Snack		
Lunch		
Snack		
Dinner		
Snack		

*Creon should always be given with a meal or snack, if it has been more than two hours since the last dosage. Do not administer generic brands of Creon.

Medication	Dosage	Times
Prevacid/Gas		
Albuterol		
Pulmozyme		
Saline		
Multi-Vitamin		
Specialty Vitamin		
Oral Antibiotic		
Inhale Antibiotic		
Nasal Spray		
Miralax		

Daily Activity

Special dietary needs:

_____

_____

_____

_____

Exercise: _____

	None	Light	Medium	Severe
Cough				
Sputum				

Stools # Daily _____ **Greasy, Yes/NO Color:** _____

Compression vest frequency: _____

Compression vest settings:

Intervals	Duration	Speed
1		
2		
3		

Pep Device frequency: _____

Additional Notes:

_____

_____

_____

_____

_____

Date: _____

Dispensed Medications:

Creon _____mg # with meals _____ # with snacks_____

	Dosage	Time
Breakfast		
Snack		
Lunch		
Snack		
Dinner		
Snack		

*Creon should always be given with a meal or snack, if it has been more than two hours since the last dosage. Do not administer generic brands of Creon.

Medication	Dosage	Times
Prevacid/Gas		
Albuterol		
Pulmozyme		
Saline		
Multi-Vitamin		
Specialty Vitamin		
Oral Antibiotic		
Inhale Antibiotic		
Nasal Spray		
Miralax		

Daily Activity

Special dietary needs:

_____

_____

_____

_____

Exercise: _____

	None	Light	Medium	Severe
Cough				
Sputum				

Stools # Daily _____ **Greasy, Yes/NO Color:** _____

Compression vest frequency: _____

Compression vest settings:

Intervals	Duration	Speed
1		
2		
3		

Pep Device frequency: _____

Additional Notes:

_____

_____

_____

_____

_____

Date: _____

Dispensed Medications:

Creon _____mg # with meals _____ # with snacks_____

	Dosage	Time
Breakfast		
Snack		
Lunch		
Snack		
Dinner		
Snack		

*Creon should always be given with a meal or snack, if it has been more than two hours since the last dosage. Do not administer generic brands of Creon.

Medication	Dosage	Times
Prevacid/Gas		
Albuterol		
Pulmozyme		
Saline		
Multi-Vitamin		
Specialty Vitamin		
Oral Antibiotic		
Inhale Antibiotic		
Nasal Spray		
Miralax		

Daily Activity

Special dietary needs:

_____

_____

_____

_____

Exercise: _____

	None	Light	Medium	Severe
Cough				
Sputum				

Stools # Daily _____ **Greasy, Yes/NO Color:** _____

Compression vest frequency: _____

Compression vest settings:

Intervals	Duration	Speed
1		
2		
3		

Pep Device frequency: _____

Additional Notes:

_____

_____

_____

_____

_____

Date: _____

Dispensed Medications:

Creon _____mg # with meals _____ # with snacks_____

	Dosage	Time
Breakfast		
Snack		
Lunch		
Snack		
Dinner		
Snack		

*Creon should always be given with a meal or snack, if it has been more than two hours since the last dosage. Do not administer generic brands of Creon.

Medication	Dosage	Times
Prevacid/Gas		
Albuterol		
Pulmozyme		
Saline		
Multi-Vitamin		
Specialty Vitamin		
Oral Antibiotic		
Inhale Antibiotic		
Nasal Spray		
Miralax		

Daily Activity

Special dietary needs:

_____

_____

_____

_____

Exercise: _____

	None	Light	Medium	Severe
Cough				
Sputum				

Stools # Daily _____ **Greasy, Yes/NO Color:** _____

Compression vest frequency: _____

Compression vest settings:

Intervals	Duration	Speed
1		
2		
3		

Pep Device frequency: _____

Additional Notes:

_____

_____

_____

_____

_____

Date: _____

Dispensed Medications:

Creon _____ mg # with meals _____ # with snacks _____

	Dosage	Time
Breakfast		
Snack		
Lunch		
Snack		
Dinner		
Snack		

*Creon should always be given with a meal or snack, if it has been more than two hours since the last dosage. Do not administer generic brands of Creon.

Medication	Dosage	Times
Prevacid/Gas		
Albuterol		
Pulmozyme		
Saline		
Multi-Vitamin		
Specialty Vitamin		
Oral Antibiotic		
Inhale Antibiotic		
Nasal Spray		
Miralax		

Daily Activity

Special dietary needs:

_____

_____

_____

_____

Exercise: _____

	None	Light	Medium	Severe
Cough				
Sputum				

Stools # Daily _____ **Greasy, Yes/NO Color:** _____

Compression vest frequency: _____

Compression vest settings:

Intervals	Duration	Speed
1		
2		
3		

Pep Device frequency: _____

Additional Notes:

_____

_____

_____

_____

_____

Date: _____

Dispensed Medications:

Creon _____ mg # with meals _____ # with snacks _____

	Dosage	Time
Breakfast		
Snack		
Lunch		
Snack		
Dinner		
Snack		

*Creon should always be given with a meal or snack, if it has been more than two hours since the last dosage. Do not administer generic brands of Creon.

Medication	Dosage	Times
Prevacid/Gas		
Albuterol		
Pulmozyme		
Saline		
Multi-Vitamin		
Specialty Vitamin		
Oral Antibiotic		
Inhale Antibiotic		
Nasal Spray		
Miralax		

Daily Activity

Special dietary needs:

_____

_____

_____

_____

Exercise: _____

	None	Light	Medium	Severe
Cough				
Sputum				

Stools # Daily _____ **Greasy, Yes/NO Color:** _____

Compression vest frequency: _____

Compression vest settings:

Intervals	Duration	Speed
1		
2		
3		

Pep Device frequency: _____

Additional Notes:

_____

_____

_____

_____

_____

Date: _____

Dispensed Medications:

Creon _____ mg # with meals _____ # with snacks _____

	Dosage	Time
Breakfast		
Snack		
Lunch		
Snack		
Dinner		
Snack		

*Creon should always be given with a meal or snack, if it has been more than two hours since the last dosage. Do not administer generic brands of Creon.

Medication	Dosage	Times
Prevacid/Gas		
Albuterol		
Pulmozyme		
Saline		
Multi-Vitamin		
Specialty Vitamin		
Oral Antibiotic		
Inhale Antibiotic		
Nasal Spray		
Miralax		

Daily Activity

Special dietary needs:
_____
_____
_____
_____

Exercise: _____

	None	Light	Medium	Severe
Cough				
Sputum				

Stools # Daily _____ **Greasy, Yes/NO Color:** _____

Compression vest frequency: _____

Compression vest settings:

Intervals	Duration	Speed
1		
2		
3		

Pep Device frequency: _____

Additional Notes:
_____
_____
_____
_____
_____

Date: _____

Dispensed Medications:

Creon _____ mg # with meals _____ # with snacks _____

	Dosage	Time
Breakfast		
Snack		
Lunch		
Snack		
Dinner		
Snack		

*Creon should always be given with a meal or snack, if it has been more than two hours since the last dosage. Do not administer generic brands of Creon.

Medication	Dosage	Times
Prevacid/Gas		
Albuterol		
Pulmozyme		
Saline		
Multi-Vitamin		
Specialty Vitamin		
Oral Antibiotic		
Inhale Antibiotic		
Nasal Spray		
Miralax		

Daily Activity

Special dietary needs:

_____

_____

_____

_____

Exercise: _____

	None	Light	Medium	Severe
Cough				
Sputum				

Stools # Daily _____ **Greasy, Yes/NO Color:** _____

Compression vest frequency: _____

Compression vest settings:

Intervals	Duration	Speed
1		
2		
3		

Pep Device frequency: _____

Additional Notes:

_____

_____

_____

_____

_____

Date: _____

Dispensed Medications:

Creon _____ mg # with meals _____ # with snacks_____

	Dosage	Time
Breakfast		
Snack		
Lunch		
Snack		
Dinner		
Snack		

*Creon should always be given with a meal or snack, if it has been more than two hours since the last dosage. Do not administer generic brands of Creon.

Medication	Dosage	Times
Prevacid/Gas		
Albuterol		
Pulmozyme		
Saline		
Multi-Vitamin		
Specialty Vitamin		
Oral Antibiotic		
Inhale Antibiotic		
Nasal Spray		
Miralax		

Daily Activity

Special dietary needs:

_____

_____

_____

_____

Exercise: _____

	None	Light	Medium	Severe
Cough				
Sputum				

Stools # Daily _____ **Greasy, Yes/NO Color:** _____

Compression vest frequency: _____

Compression vest settings:

Intervals	Duration	Speed
1		
2		
3		

Pep Device frequency: _____

Additional Notes:

_____

_____

_____

_____

_____

Date: _____

Dispensed Medications:

Creon _____mg # with meals _____ # with snacks_____

	Dosage	Time
Breakfast		
Snack		
Lunch		
Snack		
Dinner		
Snack		

*Creon should always be given with a meal or snack, if it has been more than two hours since the last dosage. Do not administer generic brands of Creon.

Medication	Dosage	Times
Prevacid/Gas		
Albuterol		
Pulmozyme		
Saline		
Multi-Vitamin		
Specialty Vitamin		
Oral Antibiotic		
Inhale Antibiotic		
Nasal Spray		
Miralax		

Daily Activity

Special dietary needs:

_____

_____

_____

_____

Exercise: _____

	None	Light	Medium	Severe
Cough				
Sputum				

Stools # Daily _____ **Greasy, Yes/NO Color:** _____

Compression vest frequency: _____

Compression vest settings:

Intervals	Duration	Speed
1		
2		
3		

Pep Device frequency: _____

Additional Notes:

_____

_____

_____

_____

_____

Date: _____

Dispensed Medications:

Creon _____ mg # with meals _____ # with snacks _____

	Dosage	Time
Breakfast		
Snack		
Lunch		
Snack		
Dinner		
Snack		

*Creon should always be given with a meal or snack, if it has been more than two hours since the last dosage. Do not administer generic brands of Creon.

Medication	Dosage	Times
Prevacid/Gas		
Albuterol		
Pulmozyme		
Saline		
Multi-Vitamin		
Specialty Vitamin		
Oral Antibiotic		
Inhale Antibiotic		
Nasal Spray		
Miralax		

Daily Activity

Special dietary needs:

_____

_____

_____

_____

Exercise: _____

	None	Light	Medium	Severe
Cough				
Sputum				

Stools # Daily _____ **Greasy, Yes/NO Color:** _____

Compression vest frequency: _____

Compression vest settings:

Intervals	Duration	Speed
1		
2		
3		

Pep Device frequency: _____

Additional Notes:

_____

_____

_____

_____

_____

Date: _____

Dispensed Medications:

Creon _____ mg # with meals _____ # with snacks _____

	Dosage	Time
Breakfast		
Snack		
Lunch		
Snack		
Dinner		
Snack		

*Creon should always be given with a meal or snack, if it has been more than two hours since the last dosage. Do not administer generic brands of Creon.

Medication	Dosage	Times
Prevacid/Gas		
Albuterol		
Pulmozyme		
Saline		
Multi-Vitamin		
Specialty Vitamin		
Oral Antibiotic		
Inhale Antibiotic		
Nasal Spray		
Miralax		

Daily Activity

Special dietary needs:

_____

_____

_____

_____

Exercise: _____

	None	Light	Medium	Severe
Cough				
Sputum				

Stools # Daily _____ **Greasy, Yes/NO Color:** _____

Compression vest frequency: _____

Compression vest settings:

Intervals	Duration	Speed
1		
2		
3		

Pep Device frequency: _____

Additional Notes:

_____

_____

_____

_____

_____

Date: _____

Dispensed Medications:

Creon _____mg # with meals _____ # with snacks_____

	Dosage	Time
Breakfast		
Snack		
Lunch		
Snack		
Dinner		
Snack		

*Creon should always be given with a meal or snack, if it has been more than two hours since the last dosage. Do not administer generic brands of Creon.

Medication	Dosage	Times
Prevacid/Gas		
Albuterol		
Pulmozyme		
Saline		
Multi-Vitamin		
Specialty Vitamin		
Oral Antibiotic		
Inhale Antibiotic		
Nasal Spray		
Miralax		

Daily Activity

Special dietary needs:

_____

_____

_____

_____

Exercise: _____

	None	Light	Medium	Severe
Cough				
Sputum				

Stools # Daily _____ **Greasy, Yes/NO Color:** _____

Compression vest frequency: _____

Compression vest settings:

Intervals	Duration	Speed
1		
2		
3		

Pep Device frequency: _____

Additional Notes:

_____

_____

_____

_____

_____

Date: _____

Dispensed Medications:

Creon _____mg # with meals _____ # with snacks_____

	Dosage	Time
Breakfast		
Snack		
Lunch		
Snack		
Dinner		
Snack		

*Creon should always be given with a meal or snack, if it has been more than two hours since the last dosage. Do not administer generic brands of Creon.

Medication	Dosage	Times
Prevacid/Gas		
Albuterol		
Pulmozyme		
Saline		
Multi-Vitamin		
Specialty Vitamin		
Oral Antibiotic		
Inhale Antibiotic		
Nasal Spray		
Miralax		

Daily Activity

Special dietary needs:

_____

_____

_____

_____

Exercise: _____

	None	Light	Medium	Severe
Cough				
Sputum				

Stools # Daily _____ **Greasy, Yes/NO   Color:** _____

Compression vest frequency: _____

Compression vest settings:

Intervals	Duration	Speed
1		
2		
3		

Pep Device frequency: _____

Additional Notes:

_____

_____

_____

_____

_____

Date: _____

Dispensed Medications:

Creon _____mg # with meals _____ # with snacks_____

	Dosage	Time
Breakfast		
Snack		
Lunch		
Snack		
Dinner		
Snack		

*Creon should always be given with a meal or snack, if it has been more than two hours since the last dosage. Do not administer generic brands of Creon.

Medication	Dosage	Times
Prevacid/Gas		
Albuterol		
Pulmozyme		
Saline		
Multi-Vitamin		
Specialty Vitamin		
Oral Antibiotic		
Inhale Antibiotic		
Nasal Spray		
Miralax		

Daily Activity

Special dietary needs:

_____
_____
_____
_____

Exercise: _____

	None	Light	Medium	Severe
Cough				
Sputum				

Stools # Daily _____ **Greasy, Yes/NO Color:** _____

Compression vest frequency: _____

Compression vest settings:

Intervals	Duration	Speed
1		
2		
3		

Pep Device frequency: _____

Additional Notes:

_____
_____
_____
_____
_____

Date: _____

Dispensed Medications:

Creon _____mg # with meals _____ # with snacks_____

	Dosage	Time
Breakfast		
Snack		
Lunch		
Snack		
Dinner		
Snack		

*Creon should always be given with a meal or snack, if it has been more than two hours since the last dosage. Do not administer generic brands of Creon.

Medication	Dosage	Times
Prevacid/Gas		
Albuterol		
Pulmozyme		
Saline		
Multi-Vitamin		
Specialty Vitamin		
Oral Antibiotic		
Inhale Antibiotic		
Nasal Spray		
Miralax		

Daily Activity

Special dietary needs:

_____

_____

_____

_____

Exercise: _____

	None	Light	Medium	Severe
Cough				
Sputum				

Stools # Daily _____ **Greasy, Yes/NO Color:** _____

Compression vest frequency: _____

Compression vest settings:

Intervals	Duration	Speed
1		
2		
3		

Pep Device frequency: _____

Additional Notes:

_____

_____

_____

_____

_____

Date: _____

Dispensed Medications:

Creon _____mg # with meals _____ # with snacks_____

	Dosage	Time
Breakfast		
Snack		
Lunch		
Snack		
Dinner		
Snack		

*Creon should always be given with a meal or snack, if it has been more than two hours since the last dosage. Do not administer generic brands of Creon.

Medication	Dosage	Times
Prevacid/Gas		
Albuterol		
Pulmozyme		
Saline		
Multi-Vitamin		
Specialty Vitamin		
Oral Antibiotic		
Inhale Antibiotic		
Nasal Spray		
Miralax		

Daily Activity

Special dietary needs:

_____

_____

_____

_____

Exercise: _____

	None	Light	Medium	Severe
Cough				
Sputum				

Stools # Daily _____ **Greasy, Yes/NO Color:** _____

Compression vest frequency: _____

Compression vest settings:

Intervals	Duration	Speed
1		
2		
3		

Pep Device frequency: _____

Additional Notes:

_____

_____

_____

_____

_____

Date: _____

Dispensed Medications:

Creon _____mg # with meals _____ # with snacks_____

	Dosage	Time
Breakfast		
Snack		
Lunch		
Snack		
Dinner		
Snack		

*Creon should always be given with a meal or snack, if it has been more than two hours since the last dosage. Do not administer generic brands of Creon.

Medication	Dosage	Times
Prevacid/Gas		
Albuterol		
Pulmozyme		
Saline		
Multi-Vitamin		
Specialty Vitamin		
Oral Antibiotic		
Inhale Antibiotic		
Nasal Spray		
Miralax		

Daily Activity

Special dietary needs:

_____

_____

_____

_____

Exercise: _____

	None	Light	Medium	Severe
Cough				
Sputum				

Stools # Daily _____   **Greasy, Yes/NO Color:** _____

Compression vest frequency: _____

Compression vest settings:

Intervals	Duration	Speed
1		
2		
3		

Pep Device frequency: _____

Additional Notes:

_____

_____

_____

_____

_____

Date: _____

Dispensed Medications:

Creon _____mg # with meals _____ # with snacks_____

	Dosage	Time
Breakfast		
Snack		
Lunch		
Snack		
Dinner		
Snack		

*Creon should always be given with a meal or snack, if it has been more than two hours since the last dosage. Do not administer generic brands of Creon.

Medication	Dosage	Times
Prevacid/Gas		
Albuterol		
Pulmozyme		
Saline		
Multi-Vitamin		
Specialty Vitamin		
Oral Antibiotic		
Inhale Antibiotic		
Nasal Spray		
Miralax		

Daily Activity

Special dietary needs:

_____

_____

_____

_____

Exercise: _____

	None	Light	Medium	Severe
Cough				
Sputum				

Stools # Daily _____ **Greasy, Yes/NO Color:** _____

Compression vest frequency: _____

Compression vest settings:

Intervals	Duration	Speed
1		
2		
3		

Pep Device frequency: _____

Additional Notes:

_____

_____

_____

_____

_____

Date: _____

Dispensed Medications:

Creon _____mg # with meals _____ # with snacks_____

	Dosage	Time
Breakfast		
Snack		
Lunch		
Snack		
Dinner		
Snack		

*Creon should always be given with a meal or snack, if it has been more than two hours since the last dosage. Do not administer generic brands of Creon.

Medication	Dosage	Times
Prevacid/Gas		
Albuterol		
Pulmozyme		
Saline		
Multi-Vitamin		
Specialty Vitamin		
Oral Antibiotic		
Inhale Antibiotic		
Nasal Spray		
Miralax		

Daily Activity

Special dietary needs:

_____

_____

_____

_____

Exercise: _____

	None	Light	Medium	Severe
Cough				
Sputum				

Stools # Daily _____ **Greasy, Yes/NO Color:** _____

Compression vest frequency: _____

Compression vest settings:

Intervals	Duration	Speed
1		
2		
3		

Pep Device frequency: _____

Additional Notes:

_____

_____

_____

_____

_____

Date: _____

Dispensed Medications:

Creon _____ mg # with meals _____ # with snacks _____

	Dosage	Time
Breakfast		
Snack		
Lunch		
Snack		
Dinner		
Snack		

*Creon should always be given with a meal or snack, if it has been more than two hours since the last dosage. Do not administer generic brands of Creon.

Medication	Dosage	Times
Prevacid/Gas		
Albuterol		
Pulmozyme		
Saline		
Multi-Vitamin		
Specialty Vitamin		
Oral Antibiotic		
Inhale Antibiotic		
Nasal Spray		
Miralax		

Daily Activity

Special dietary needs:

_____

_____

_____

_____

Exercise: _____

	None	Light	Medium	Severe
Cough				
Sputum				

Stools # Daily _____ **Greasy, Yes/NO Color:** _____

Compression vest frequency: _____

Compression vest settings:

Intervals	Duration	Speed
1		
2		
3		

Pep Device frequency: _____

Additional Notes:

_____

_____

_____

_____

_____

Date: _____

Dispensed Medications:

Creon _____mg # with meals _____ # with snacks_____

	Dosage	Time
Breakfast		
Snack		
Lunch		
Snack		
Dinner		
Snack		

*Creon should always be given with a meal or snack, if it has been more than two hours since the last dosage. Do not administer generic brands of Creon.

Medication	Dosage	Times
Prevacid/Gas		
Albuterol		
Pulmozyme		
Saline		
Multi-Vitamin		
Specialty Vitamin		
Oral Antibiotic		
Inhale Antibiotic		
Nasal Spray		
Miralax		

Daily Activity

Special dietary needs:

_____
_____
_____
_____

Exercise: _____

	None	Light	Medium	Severe
Cough				
Sputum				

Stools # Daily _____ **Greasy, Yes/NO Color:** _____

Compression vest frequency: _____

Compression vest settings:

Intervals	Duration	Speed
1		
2		
3		

Pep Device frequency: _____

Additional Notes:

_____
_____
_____
_____
_____

Date: _____

Dispensed Medications:

Creon _____ mg # with meals _____ # with snacks _____

	Dosage	Time
Breakfast		
Snack		
Lunch		
Snack		
Dinner		
Snack		

*Creon should always be given with a meal or snack, if it has been more than two hours since the last dosage. Do not administer generic brands of Creon.

Medication	Dosage	Times
Prevacid/Gas		
Albuterol		
Pulmozyme		
Saline		
Multi-Vitamin		
Specialty Vitamin		
Oral Antibiotic		
Inhale Antibiotic		
Nasal Spray		
Miralax		

Daily Activity

Special dietary needs:

_____

_____

_____

_____

Exercise: _____

	None	Light	Medium	Severe
Cough				
Sputum				

Stools # Daily _____ **Greasy, Yes/NO Color:** _____

Compression vest frequency: _____

Compression vest settings:

Intervals	Duration	Speed
1		
2		
3		

Pep Device frequency: _____

Additional Notes:

_____

_____

_____

_____

_____

Date: _____

Dispensed Medications:

Creon _____ mg # with meals _____ # with snacks _____

	Dosage	Time
Breakfast		
Snack		
Lunch		
Snack		
Dinner		
Snack		

*Creon should always be given with a meal or snack, if it has been more than two hours since the last dosage. Do not administer generic brands of Creon.

Medication	Dosage	Times
Prevacid/Gas		
Albuterol		
Pulmozyme		
Saline		
Multi-Vitamin		
Specialty Vitamin		
Oral Antibiotic		
Inhale Antibiotic		
Nasal Spray		
Miralax		

Daily Activity

Special dietary needs:
_____
_____
_____
_____

Exercise: _____

	None	Light	Medium	Severe
Cough				
Sputum				

Stools # Daily _____ **Greasy, Yes/NO Color:** _____

Compression vest frequency: _____

Compression vest settings:

Intervals	Duration	Speed
1		
2		
3		

Pep Device frequency: _____

Additional Notes:
_____
_____
_____
_____
_____

Date: _____

Dispensed Medications:

Creon _____mg # with meals _____ # with snacks_____

	Dosage	Time
Breakfast		
Snack		
Lunch		
Snack		
Dinner		
Snack		

*Creon should always be given with a meal or snack, if it has been more than two hours since the last dosage. Do not administer generic brands of Creon.

Medication	Dosage	Times
Prevacid/Gas		
Albuterol		
Pulmozyme		
Saline		
Multi-Vitamin		
Specialty Vitamin		
Oral Antibiotic		
Inhale Antibiotic		
Nasal Spray		
Miralax		

Daily Activity

Special dietary needs:

_____

_____

_____

_____

Exercise: _____

	None	Light	Medium	Severe
Cough				
Sputum				

Stools # Daily _____ **Greasy, Yes/NO Color:** _____

Compression vest frequency: _____

Compression vest settings:

Intervals	Duration	Speed
1		
2		
3		

Pep Device frequency: _____

Additional Notes:

_____

_____

_____

_____

_____

Date: _____

Dispensed Medications:

Creon _____mg # with meals _____ # with snacks_____

	Dosage	Time
Breakfast		
Snack		
Lunch		
Snack		
Dinner		
Snack		

*Creon should always be given with a meal or snack, if it has been more than two hours since the last dosage. Do not administer generic brands of Creon.

Medication	Dosage	Times
Prevacid/Gas		
Albuterol		
Pulmozyme		
Saline		
Multi-Vitamin		
Specialty Vitamin		
Oral Antibiotic		
Inhale Antibiotic		
Nasal Spray		
Miralax		

Daily Activity

Special dietary needs:

_____

_____

_____

_____

Exercise: _____

	None	Light	Medium	Severe
Cough				
Sputum				

Stools # Daily _____ **Greasy, Yes/NO Color:** _____

Compression vest frequency: _____

Compression vest settings:

Intervals	Duration	Speed
1		
2		
3		

Pep Device frequency: _____

Additional Notes:

_____

_____

_____

_____

_____

Date: _____

Dispensed Medications:

Creon _____mg # with meals _____ # with snacks_____

	Dosage	Time
Breakfast		
Snack		
Lunch		
Snack		
Dinner		
Snack		

*Creon should always be given with a meal or snack, if it has been more than two hours since the last dosage. Do not administer generic brands of Creon.

Medication	Dosage	Times
Prevacid/Gas		
Albuterol		
Pulmozyme		
Saline		
Multi-Vitamin		
Specialty Vitamin		
Oral Antibiotic		
Inhale Antibiotic		
Nasal Spray		
Miralax		

Daily Activity

Special dietary needs:

_____

_____

_____

_____

Exercise: _____

	None	Light	Medium	Severe
Cough				
Sputum				

Stools # Daily _____ **Greasy, Yes/NO Color:** _____

Compression vest frequency: _____

Compression vest settings:

Intervals	Duration	Speed
1		
2		
3		

Pep Device frequency: _____

Additional Notes:

_____

_____

_____

_____

_____

Date: _____

Dispensed Medications:

Creon _____ mg # with meals _____ # with snacks _____

	Dosage	Time
Breakfast		
Snack		
Lunch		
Snack		
Dinner		
Snack		

*Creon should always be given with a meal or snack, if it has been more than two hours since the last dosage. Do not administer generic brands of Creon.

Medication	Dosage	Times
Prevacid/Gas		
Albuterol		
Pulmozyme		
Saline		
Multi-Vitamin		
Specialty Vitamin		
Oral Antibiotic		
Inhale Antibiotic		
Nasal Spray		
Miralax		

Daily Activity

Special dietary needs:

_____
_____
_____
_____

Exercise: _____

	None	Light	Medium	Severe
Cough				
Sputum				

Stools # Daily _____ **Greasy, Yes/NO Color:** _____

Compression vest frequency: _____

Compression vest settings:

Intervals	Duration	Speed
1		
2		
3		

Pep Device frequency: _____

Additional Notes:

_____
_____
_____
_____
_____

Date: _____

Dispensed Medications:

Creon _____mg # with meals _____ # with snacks_____

	Dosage	Time
Breakfast		
Snack		
Lunch		
Snack		
Dinner		
Snack		

*Creon should always be given with a meal or snack, if it has been more than two hours since the last dosage. Do not administer generic brands of Creon.

Medication	Dosage	Times
Prevacid/Gas		
Albuterol		
Pulmozyme		
Saline		
Multi-Vitamin		
Specialty Vitamin		
Oral Antibiotic		
Inhale Antibiotic		
Nasal Spray		
Miralax		

Daily Activity

Special dietary needs:

_____

_____

_____

_____

Exercise: _____

	None	Light	Medium	Severe
Cough				
Sputum				

Stools # Daily _____ **Greasy, Yes/NO Color:** _____

Compression vest frequency: _____

Compression vest settings:

Intervals	Duration	Speed
1		
2		
3		

Pep Device frequency: _____

Additional Notes:

_____

_____

_____

_____

Date: _____

Dispensed Medications:

Creon _____ mg # with meals _____ # with snacks _____

	Dosage	Time
Breakfast		
Snack		
Lunch		
Snack		
Dinner		
Snack		

*Creon should always be given with a meal or snack, if it has been more than two hours since the last dosage. Do not administer generic brands of Creon.

Medication	Dosage	Times
Prevacid/Gas		
Albuterol		
Pulmozyme		
Saline		
Multi-Vitamin		
Specialty Vitamin		
Oral Antibiotic		
Inhale Antibiotic		
Nasal Spray		
Miralax		

Daily Activity

Special dietary needs:

_____

_____

_____

_____

Exercise: _____

	None	Light	Medium	Severe
Cough				
Sputum				

Stools # Daily _____ **Greasy, Yes/NO Color:** _____

Compression vest frequency: _____

Compression vest settings:

Intervals	Duration	Speed
1		
2		
3		

Pep Device frequency: _____

Additional Notes:

_____

_____

_____

_____

Date: _____

Dispensed Medications:

Creon _____mg # with meals _____ # with snacks_____

	Dosage	Time
Breakfast		
Snack		
Lunch		
Snack		
Dinner		
Snack		

*Creon should always be given with a meal or snack, if it has been more than two hours since the last dosage. Do not administer generic brands of Creon.

Medication	Dosage	Times
Prevacid/Gas		
Albuterol		
Pulmozyme		
Saline		
Multi-Vitamin		
Specialty Vitamin		
Oral Antibiotic		
Inhale Antibiotic		
Nasal Spray		
Miralax		

Daily Activity

Special dietary needs:

_____

_____

_____

_____

Exercise: _____

	None	Light	Medium	Severe
Cough				
Sputum				

Stools # Daily _____ **Greasy, Yes/NO Color:** _____

Compression vest frequency: _____

Compression vest settings:

Intervals	Duration	Speed
1		
2		
3		

Pep Device frequency: _____

Additional Notes:

_____

_____

_____

_____

_____

Date: _____

Dispensed Medications:

Creon _____ mg # with meals _____ # with snacks _____

	Dosage	Time
Breakfast		
Snack		
Lunch		
Snack		
Dinner		
Snack		

*Creon should always be given with a meal or snack, if it has been more than two hours since the last dosage. Do not administer generic brands of Creon.

Medication	Dosage	Times
Prevacid/Gas		
Albuterol		
Pulmozyme		
Saline		
Multi-Vitamin		
Specialty Vitamin		
Oral Antibiotic		
Inhale Antibiotic		
Nasal Spray		
Miralax		

Daily Activity

Special dietary needs:

_____
_____
_____
_____

Exercise: _____

	None	Light	Medium	Severe
Cough				
Sputum				

Stools # Daily _____ **Greasy, Yes/NO Color:** _____

Compression vest frequency: _____

Compression vest settings:

Intervals	Duration	Speed
1		
2		
3		

Pep Device frequency: _____

Additional Notes:

_____
_____
_____
_____

Date: _____

Dispensed Medications:

Creon _____ mg # with meals _____ # with snacks _____

	Dosage	Time
Breakfast		
Snack		
Lunch		
Snack		
Dinner		
Snack		

*Creon should always be given with a meal or snack, if it has been more than two hours since the last dosage. Do not administer generic brands of Creon.

Medication	Dosage	Times
Prevacid/Gas		
Albuterol		
Pulmozyme		
Saline		
Multi-Vitamin		
Specialty Vitamin		
Oral Antibiotic		
Inhale Antibiotic		
Nasal Spray		
Miralax		

Daily Activity

Special dietary needs:

_____

_____

_____

_____

Exercise: _____

	None	Light	Medium	Severe
Cough				
Sputum				

Stools # Daily _____ **Greasy, Yes/NO Color:** _____

Compression vest frequency: _____

Compression vest settings:

Intervals	Duration	Speed
1		
2		
3		

Pep Device frequency: _____

Additional Notes:

_____

_____

_____

_____

_____

Date: _____

Dispensed Medications:

Creon _____mg # with meals _____ # with snacks_____

	Dosage	Time
Breakfast		
Snack		
Lunch		
Snack		
Dinner		
Snack		

*Creon should always be given with a meal or snack, if it has been more than two hours since the last dosage. Do not administer generic brands of Creon.

Medication	Dosage	Times
Prevacid/Gas		
Albuterol		
Pulmozyme		
Saline		
Multi-Vitamin		
Specialty Vitamin		
Oral Antibiotic		
Inhale Antibiotic		
Nasal Spray		
Miralax		

Daily Activity

Special dietary needs:

_____
_____
_____
_____

Exercise: _____

	None	Light	Medium	Severe
Cough				
Sputum				

Stools # Daily _____ **Greasy, Yes/NO Color:** _____

Compression vest frequency: _____

Compression vest settings:

Intervals	Duration	Speed
1		
2		
3		

Pep Device frequency: _____

Additional Notes:

_____
_____
_____
_____
_____

Date: _____

Dispensed Medications:

Creon _____ mg # with meals _____ # with snacks _____

	Dosage	Time
Breakfast		
Snack		
Lunch		
Snack		
Dinner		
Snack		

*Creon should always be given with a meal or snack, if it has been more than two hours since the last dosage. Do not administer generic brands of Creon.

Medication	Dosage	Times
Prevacid/Gas		
Albuterol		
Pulmozyme		
Saline		
Multi-Vitamin		
Specialty Vitamin		
Oral Antibiotic		
Inhale Antibiotic		
Nasal Spray		
Miralax		

Daily Activity

Special dietary needs:

_____

_____

_____

_____

Exercise: _____

	None	Light	Medium	Severe
Cough				
Sputum				

Stools # Daily _____ **Greasy, Yes/NO Color:** _____

Compression vest frequency: _____

Compression vest settings:

Intervals	Duration	Speed
1		
2		
3		

Pep Device frequency: _____

Additional Notes:

_____

_____

_____

_____

_____

Date: _____

Dispensed Medications:

Creon _____mg # with meals _____ # with snacks_____

	Dosage	Time
Breakfast		
Snack		
Lunch		
Snack		
Dinner		
Snack		

*Creon should always be given with a meal or snack, if it has been more than two hours since the last dosage. Do not administer generic brands of Creon.

Medication	Dosage	Times
Prevacid/Gas		
Albuterol		
Pulmozyme		
Saline		
Multi-Vitamin		
Specialty Vitamin		
Oral Antibiotic		
Inhale Antibiotic		
Nasal Spray		
Miralax		

Daily Activity

Special dietary needs:

_____

_____

_____

_____

Exercise: _____

	None	Light	Medium	Severe
Cough				
Sputum				

Stools # Daily _____ **Greasy, Yes/NO Color:** _____

Compression vest frequency: _____

Compression vest settings:

Intervals	Duration	Speed
1		
2		
3		

Pep Device frequency: _____

Additional Notes:

_____

_____

_____

_____

_____

Date: _____

Dispensed Medications:

Creon _____mg # with meals _____ # with snacks_____

	Dosage	Time
Breakfast		
Snack		
Lunch		
Snack		
Dinner		
Snack		

*Creon should always be given with a meal or snack, if it has been more than two hours since the last dosage. Do not administer generic brands of Creon.

Medication	Dosage	Times
Prevacid/Gas		
Albuterol		
Pulmozyme		
Saline		
Multi-Vitamin		
Specialty Vitamin		
Oral Antibiotic		
Inhale Antibiotic		
Nasal Spray		
Miralax		

Daily Activity

Special dietary needs:

_____
_____
_____
_____

Exercise: _____

	None	Light	Medium	Severe
Cough				
Sputum				

Stools # Daily _____ **Greasy, Yes/NO Color:** _____

Compression vest frequency: _____

Compression vest settings:

Intervals	Duration	Speed
1		
2		
3		

Pep Device frequency: _____

Additional Notes:

_____
_____
_____
_____
_____

Date: _____

Dispensed Medications:

Creon _____ mg # with meals _____ # with snacks _____

	Dosage	Time
Breakfast		
Snack		
Lunch		
Snack		
Dinner		
Snack		

*Creon should always be given with a meal or snack, if it has been more than two hours since the last dosage. Do not administer generic brands of Creon.

Medication	Dosage	Times
Prevacid/Gas		
Albuterol		
Pulmozyme		
Saline		
Multi-Vitamin		
Specialty Vitamin		
Oral Antibiotic		
Inhale Antibiotic		
Nasal Spray		
Miralax		

Daily Activity

Special dietary needs:

_____

_____

_____

_____

Exercise: _____

	None	Light	Medium	Severe
Cough				
Sputum				

Stools # Daily _____ **Greasy, Yes/NO Color:** _____

Compression vest frequency: _____

Compression vest settings:

Intervals	Duration	Speed
1		
2		
3		

Pep Device frequency: _____

Additional Notes:

_____

_____

_____

_____

_____

Date: _____

Dispensed Medications:

Creon _____ mg # with meals _____ # with snacks_____

	Dosage	Time
Breakfast		
Snack		
Lunch		
Snack		
Dinner		
Snack		

*Creon should always be given with a meal or snack, if it has been more than two hours since the last dosage. Do not administer generic brands of Creon.

Medication	Dosage	Times
Prevacid/Gas		
Albuterol		
Pulmozyme		
Saline		
Multi-Vitamin		
Specialty Vitamin		
Oral Antibiotic		
Inhale Antibiotic		
Nasal Spray		
Miralax		

Daily Activity

Special dietary needs:

_____

_____

_____

_____

Exercise: _____

	None	Light	Medium	Severe
Cough				
Sputum				

Stools # Daily _____ **Greasy, Yes/NO Color:** _____

Compression vest frequency: _____

Compression vest settings:

Intervals	Duration	Speed
1		
2		
3		

Pep Device frequency: _____

Additional Notes:

_____

_____

_____

_____

_____

Date: _____

Dispensed Medications:

Creon _____mg # with meals _____ # with snacks_____

	Dosage	Time
Breakfast		
Snack		
Lunch		
Snack		
Dinner		
Snack		

*Creon should always be given with a meal or snack, if it has been more than two hours since the last dosage. Do not administer generic brands of Creon.

Medication	Dosage	Times
Prevacid/Gas		
Albuterol		
Pulmozyme		
Saline		
Multi-Vitamin		
Specialty Vitamin		
Oral Antibiotic		
Inhale Antibiotic		
Nasal Spray		
Miralax		

Daily Activity

Special dietary needs:

_____

_____

_____

_____

Exercise: _____

	None	Light	Medium	Severe
Cough				
Sputum				

Stools # Daily _____ **Greasy, Yes/NO Color:** _____

Compression vest frequency: _____

Compression vest settings:

Intervals	Duration	Speed
1		
2		
3		

Pep Device frequency: _____

Additional Notes:

_____

_____

_____

_____

Date: _____

Dispensed Medications:

Creon _____ mg # with meals _____ # with snacks _____

	Dosage	Time
Breakfast		
Snack		
Lunch		
Snack		
Dinner		
Snack		

*Creon should always be given with a meal or snack, if it has been more than two hours since the last dosage. Do not administer generic brands of Creon.

Medication	Dosage	Times
Prevacid/Gas		
Albuterol		
Pulmozyme		
Saline		
Multi-Vitamin		
Specialty Vitamin		
Oral Antibiotic		
Inhale Antibiotic		
Nasal Spray		
Miralax		

Daily Activity

Special dietary needs:

_____

_____

_____

_____

Exercise: _____

	None	Light	Medium	Severe
Cough				
Sputum				

Stools # Daily _____ **Greasy, Yes/NO Color:** _____

Compression vest frequency: _____

Compression vest settings:

Intervals	Duration	Speed
1		
2		
3		

Pep Device frequency: _____

Additional Notes:

_____

_____

_____

_____

_____

Date: _____

Dispensed Medications:

Creon _____mg # with meals _____ # with snacks_____

	Dosage	Time
Breakfast		
Snack		
Lunch		
Snack		
Dinner		
Snack		

*Creon should always be given with a meal or snack, if it has been more than two hours since the last dosage. Do not administer generic brands of Creon.

Medication	Dosage	Times
Prevacid/Gas		
Albuterol		
Pulmozyme		
Saline		
Multi-Vitamin		
Specialty Vitamin		
Oral Antibiotic		
Inhale Antibiotic		
Nasal Spray		
Miralax		

Daily Activity

Special dietary needs:

_____
_____
_____
_____

Exercise: _____

	None	Light	Medium	Severe
Cough				
Sputum				

Stools # Daily _____ **Greasy, Yes/NO Color:** _____

Compression vest frequency: _____

Compression vest settings:

Intervals	Duration	Speed
1		
2		
3		

Pep Device frequency: _____

Additional Notes:

_____
_____
_____
_____
_____

Date: _____

Dispensed Medications:

Creon _____mg # with meals _____ # with snacks_____

	Dosage	Time
Breakfast		
Snack		
Lunch		
Snack		
Dinner		
Snack		

*Creon should always be given with a meal or snack, if it has been more than two hours since the last dosage. Do not administer generic brands of Creon.

Medication	Dosage	Times
Prevacid/Gas		
Albuterol		
Pulmozyme		
Saline		
Multi-Vitamin		
Specialty Vitamin		
Oral Antibiotic		
Inhale Antibiotic		
Nasal Spray		
Miralax		

Daily Activity

Special dietary needs:

_____
_____
_____
_____

Exercise: _____

	None	Light	Medium	Severe
Cough				
Sputum				

Stools # Daily _____ **Greasy, Yes/NO Color:** _____

Compression vest frequency: _____

Compression vest settings:

Intervals	Duration	Speed
1		
2		
3		

Pep Device frequency: _____

Additional Notes:

_____
_____
_____
_____
_____

Date: _____

Dispensed Medications:

Creon _____ mg # with meals _____ # with snacks _____

	Dosage	Time
Breakfast		
Snack		
Lunch		
Snack		
Dinner		
Snack		

*Creon should always be given with a meal or snack, if it has been more than two hours since the last dosage. Do not administer generic brands of Creon.

Medication	Dosage	Times
Prevacid/Gas		
Albuterol		
Pulmozyme		
Saline		
Multi-Vitamin		
Specialty Vitamin		
Oral Antibiotic		
Inhale Antibiotic		
Nasal Spray		
Miralax		

Daily Activity

Special dietary needs:

_____

_____

_____

_____

Exercise: _____

	None	Light	Medium	Severe
Cough				
Sputum				

Stools # Daily _____ **Greasy, Yes/NO Color:** _____

Compression vest frequency: _____

Compression vest settings:

Intervals	Duration	Speed
1		
2		
3		

Pep Device frequency: _____

Additional Notes:

_____

_____

_____

_____

_____

Date: _____

Dispensed Medications:

Creon _____mg # with meals _____ # with snacks_____

	Dosage	Time
Breakfast		
Snack		
Lunch		
Snack		
Dinner		
Snack		

*Creon should always be given with a meal or snack, if it has been more than two hours since the last dosage. Do not administer generic brands of Creon.

Medication	Dosage	Times
Prevacid/Gas		
Albuterol		
Pulmozyme		
Saline		
Multi-Vitamin		
Specialty Vitamin		
Oral Antibiotic		
Inhale Antibiotic		
Nasal Spray		
Miralax		

Daily Activity

Special dietary needs:

_____

_____

_____

_____

Exercise: _____

	None	Light	Medium	Severe
Cough				
Sputum				

Stools # Daily _____ **Greasy, Yes/NO Color:** _____

Compression vest frequency: _____

Compression vest settings:

Intervals	Duration	Speed
1		
2		
3		

Pep Device frequency: _____

Additional Notes:

_____

_____

_____

_____

Date: _____

Dispensed Medications:

Creon _____mg # with meals _____ # with snacks_____

	Dosage	Time
Breakfast		
Snack		
Lunch		
Snack		
Dinner		
Snack		

*Creon should always be given with a meal or snack, if it has been more than two hours since the last dosage. Do not administer generic brands of Creon.

Medication	Dosage	Times
Prevacid/Gas		
Albuterol		
Pulmozyme		
Saline		
Multi-Vitamin		
Specialty Vitamin		
Oral Antibiotic		
Inhale Antibiotic		
Nasal Spray		
Miralax		

Daily Activity

Special dietary needs:
_____
_____
_____
_____

Exercise: _____

	None	Light	Medium	Severe
Cough				
Sputum				

Stools # Daily _____ Greasy, Yes/NO Color: _____

Compression vest frequency: _____

Compression vest settings:

Intervals	Duration	Speed
1		
2		
3		

Pep Device frequency: _____

Additional Notes:
_____
_____
_____
_____
_____

Date: _____

Dispensed Medications:

Creon _____mg # with meals _____ # with snacks_____

	Dosage	Time
Breakfast		
Snack		
Lunch		
Snack		
Dinner		
Snack		

*Creon should always be given with a meal or snack, if it has been more than two hours since the last dosage. Do not administer generic brands of Creon.

Medication	Dosage	Times
Prevacid/Gas		
Albuterol		
Pulmozyme		
Saline		
Multi-Vitamin		
Specialty Vitamin		
Oral Antibiotic		
Inhale Antibiotic		
Nasal Spray		
Miralax		

Daily Activity

Special dietary needs:
_____
_____
_____
_____

Exercise: _____

	None	Light	Medium	Severe
Cough				
Sputum				

Stools # Daily _____ **Greasy, Yes/NO Color:** _____

Compression vest frequency: _____

Compression vest settings:

Intervals	Duration	Speed
1		
2		
3		

Pep Device frequency: _____

Additional Notes:
_____
_____
_____
_____
_____

Date: _____

Dispensed Medications:

Creon _____mg # with meals _____ # with snacks_____

	Dosage	Time
Breakfast		
Snack		
Lunch		
Snack		
Dinner		
Snack		

*Creon should always be given with a meal or snack, if it has been more than two hours since the last dosage. Do not administer generic brands of Creon.

Medication	Dosage	Times
Prevacid/Gas		
Albuterol		
Pulmozyme		
Saline		
Multi-Vitamin		
Specialty Vitamin		
Oral Antibiotic		
Inhale Antibiotic		
Nasal Spray		
Miralax		

Daily Activity

Special dietary needs:

_____
_____
_____
_____

Exercise: _____

	None	Light	Medium	Severe
Cough				
Sputum				

Stools # Daily _____ **Greasy, Yes/NO Color:** _____

Compression vest frequency: _____

Compression vest settings:

Intervals	Duration	Speed
1		
2		
3		

Pep Device frequency: _____

Additional Notes:

_____
_____
_____
_____
_____

Date: _____

Dispensed Medications:

Creon _____mg # with meals _____ # with snacks_____

	Dosage	Time
Breakfast		
Snack		
Lunch		
Snack		
Dinner		
Snack		

*Creon should always be given with a meal or snack, if it has been more than two hours since the last dosage. Do not administer generic brands of Creon.

Medication	Dosage	Times
Prevacid/Gas		
Albuterol		
Pulmozyme		
Saline		
Multi-Vitamin		
Specialty Vitamin		
Oral Antibiotic		
Inhale Antibiotic		
Nasal Spray		
Miralax		

Daily Activity

Special dietary needs:

_____

_____

_____

_____

Exercise: _____

	None	Light	Medium	Severe
Cough				
Sputum				

Stools # Daily _____ **Greasy, Yes/NO Color:** _____

Compression vest frequency: _____

Compression vest settings:

Intervals	Duration	Speed
1		
2		
3		

Pep Device frequency: _____

Additional Notes:

_____

_____

_____

_____

_____

Date: _____

Dispensed Medications:

Creon _____mg # with meals _____ # with snacks_____

	Dosage	Time
Breakfast		
Snack		
Lunch		
Snack		
Dinner		
Snack		

*Creon should always be given with a meal or snack, if it has been more than two hours since the last dosage. Do not administer generic brands of Creon.

Medication	Dosage	Times
Prevacid/Gas		
Albuterol		
Pulmozyme		
Saline		
Multi-Vitamin		
Specialty Vitamin		
Oral Antibiotic		
Inhale Antibiotic		
Nasal Spray		
Miralax		

Daily Activity

Special dietary needs:

_____

_____

_____

_____

Exercise: _____

	None	Light	Medium	Severe
Cough				
Sputum				

Stools # Daily _____ **Greasy, Yes/NO Color:** _____

Compression vest frequency: _____

Compression vest settings:

Intervals	Duration	Speed
1		
2		
3		

Pep Device frequency: _____

Additional Notes:

_____

_____

_____

_____

_____

Date: _____

Dispensed Medications:

Creon _____ mg # with meals _____ # with snacks _____

	Dosage	Time
Breakfast		
Snack		
Lunch		
Snack		
Dinner		
Snack		

*Creon should always be given with a meal or snack, if it has been more than two hours since the last dosage. Do not administer generic brands of Creon.

Medication	Dosage	Times
Prevacid/Gas		
Albuterol		
Pulmozyme		
Saline		
Multi-Vitamin		
Specialty Vitamin		
Oral Antibiotic		
Inhale Antibiotic		
Nasal Spray		
Miralax		

Daily Activity

Special dietary needs:

_____

_____

_____

_____

Exercise: _____

	None	Light	Medium	Severe
Cough				
Sputum				

Stools # Daily _____ **Greasy, Yes/NO Color:** _____

Compression vest frequency: _____

Compression vest settings:

Intervals	Duration	Speed
1		
2		
3		

Pep Device frequency: _____

Additional Notes:

_____

_____

_____

_____

_____

Date: _____

Dispensed Medications:

Creon _____mg # with meals _____ # with snacks_____

	Dosage	Time
Breakfast		
Snack		
Lunch		
Snack		
Dinner		
Snack		

*Creon should always be given with a meal or snack, if it has been more than two hours since the last dosage. Do not administer generic brands of Creon.

Medication	Dosage	Times
Prevacid/Gas		
Albuterol		
Pulmozyme		
Saline		
Multi-Vitamin		
Specialty Vitamin		
Oral Antibiotic		
Inhale Antibiotic		
Nasal Spray		
Miralax		

Daily Activity

Special dietary needs:

_____
_____
_____
_____

Exercise: _____

	None	Light	Medium	Severe
Cough				
Sputum				

Stools # Daily _____ **Greasy, Yes/NO Color:** _____

Compression vest frequency: _____

Compression vest settings:

Intervals	Duration	Speed
1		
2		
3		

Pep Device frequency: _____

Additional Notes:

_____
_____
_____
_____
_____

Date: _____

Dispensed Medications:

Creon _____mg # with meals _____ # with snacks_____

	Dosage	Time
Breakfast		
Snack		
Lunch		
Snack		
Dinner		
Snack		

*Creon should always be given with a meal or snack, if it has been more than two hours since the last dosage. Do not administer generic brands of Creon.

Medication	Dosage	Times
Prevacid/Gas		
Albuterol		
Pulmozyme		
Saline		
Multi-Vitamin		
Specialty Vitamin		
Oral Antibiotic		
Inhale Antibiotic		
Nasal Spray		
Miralax		

Daily Activity

Special dietary needs:

_____

_____

_____

_____

Exercise: _____

	None	Light	Medium	Severe
Cough				
Sputum				

Stools # Daily _____ **Greasy, Yes/NO Color:** _____

Compression vest frequency: _____

Compression vest settings:

Intervals	Duration	Speed
1		
2		
3		

Pep Device frequency: _____

Additional Notes:

_____

_____

_____

_____

_____

Date: _____

Dispensed Medications:

Creon _____mg # with meals _____ # with snacks_____

	Dosage	Time
Breakfast		
Snack		
Lunch		
Snack		
Dinner		
Snack		

*Creon should always be given with a meal or snack, if it has been more than two hours since the last dosage. Do not administer generic brands of Creon.

Medication	Dosage	Times
Prevacid/Gas		
Albuterol		
Pulmozyme		
Saline		
Multi-Vitamin		
Specialty Vitamin		
Oral Antibiotic		
Inhale Antibiotic		
Nasal Spray		
Miralax		

Daily Activity

Special dietary needs:
_____
_____
_____
_____

Exercise: _____

	None	Light	Medium	Severe
Cough				
Sputum				

Stools # Daily _____ **Greasy, Yes/NO Color:** _____

Compression vest frequency: _____

Compression vest settings:

Intervals	Duration	Speed
1		
2		
3		

Pep Device frequency: _____

Additional Notes:
_____
_____
_____
_____
_____

Date: _____

Dispensed Medications:

Creon _____mg # with meals _____ # with snacks_____

	Dosage	Time
Breakfast		
Snack		
Lunch		
Snack		
Dinner		
Snack		

*Creon should always be given with a meal or snack, if it has been more than two hours since the last dosage. Do not administer generic brands of Creon.

Medication	Dosage	Times
Prevacid/Gas		
Albuterol		
Pulmozyme		
Saline		
Multi-Vitamin		
Specialty Vitamin		
Oral Antibiotic		
Inhale Antibiotic		
Nasal Spray		
Miralax		

Daily Activity

Special dietary needs:

_____

_____

_____

_____

Exercise: _____

	None	Light	Medium	Severe
Cough				
Sputum				

Stools # Daily _____ **Greasy, Yes/NO Color:** _____

Compression vest frequency: _____

Compression vest settings:

Intervals	Duration	Speed
1		
2		
3		

Pep Device frequency: _____

Additional Notes:

_____

_____

_____

_____

Date: _____

Dispensed Medications:

Creon _____ mg # with meals _____ # with snacks _____

	Dosage	Time
Breakfast		
Snack		
Lunch		
Snack		
Dinner		
Snack		

*Creon should always be given with a meal or snack, if it has been more than two hours since the last dosage. Do not administer generic brands of Creon.

Medication	Dosage	Times
Prevacid/Gas		
Albuterol		
Pulmozyme		
Saline		
Multi-Vitamin		
Specialty Vitamin		
Oral Antibiotic		
Inhale Antibiotic		
Nasal Spray		
Miralax		

Daily Activity

Special dietary needs:

_____

_____

_____

_____

Exercise: _____

	None	Light	Medium	Severe
Cough				
Sputum				

Stools # Daily _____ **Greasy, Yes/NO Color:** _____

Compression vest frequency: _____

Compression vest settings:

Intervals	Duration	Speed
1		
2		
3		

Pep Device frequency: _____

Additional Notes:

_____

_____

_____

_____

Date: _____

Dispensed Medications:

Creon _____ mg # with meals _____ # with snacks _____

	Dosage	Time
Breakfast		
Snack		
Lunch		
Snack		
Dinner		
Snack		

*Creon should always be given with a meal or snack, if it has been more than two hours since the last dosage. Do not administer generic brands of Creon.

Medication	Dosage	Times
Prevacid/Gas		
Albuterol		
Pulmozyme		
Saline		
Multi-Vitamin		
Specialty Vitamin		
Oral Antibiotic		
Inhale Antibiotic		
Nasal Spray		
Miralax		

Daily Activity

Special dietary needs:

_____
_____
_____
_____

Exercise: _____

	None	Light	Medium	Severe
Cough				
Sputum				

Stools # Daily _____ **Greasy, Yes/NO Color:** _____

Compression vest frequency: _____

Compression vest settings:

Intervals	Duration	Speed
1		
2		
3		

Pep Device frequency: _____

Additional Notes:

_____
_____
_____
_____
_____

Date: _____

Dispensed Medications:

Creon _____mg # with meals _____ # with snacks_____

	Dosage	Time
Breakfast		
Snack		
Lunch		
Snack		
Dinner		
Snack		

*Creon should always be given with a meal or snack, if it has been more than two hours since the last dosage. Do not administer generic brands of Creon.

Medication	Dosage	Times
Prevacid/Gas		
Albuterol		
Pulmozyme		
Saline		
Multi-Vitamin		
Specialty Vitamin		
Oral Antibiotic		
Inhale Antibiotic		
Nasal Spray		
Miralax		

Daily Activity

Special dietary needs:

_____

_____

_____

_____

Exercise: _____

	None	Light	Medium	Severe
Cough				
Sputum				

Stools # Daily _____ **Greasy, Yes/NO Color:** _____

Compression vest frequency: _____

Compression vest settings:

Intervals	Duration	Speed
1		
2		
3		

Pep Device frequency: _____

Additional Notes:

_____

_____

_____

_____

_____

Date: _____

Dispensed Medications:

Creon _____mg # with meals _____ # with snacks _____

	Dosage	Time
Breakfast		
Snack		
Lunch		
Snack		
Dinner		
Snack		

*Creon should always be given with a meal or snack, if it has been more than two hours since the last dosage. Do not administer generic brands of Creon.

Medication	Dosage	Times
Prevacid/Gas		
Albuterol		
Pulmozyme		
Saline		
Multi-Vitamin		
Specialty Vitamin		
Oral Antibiotic		
Inhale Antibiotic		
Nasal Spray		
Miralax		

Daily Activity

Special dietary needs:

_____

_____

_____

Exercise: _____

	None	Light	Medium	Severe
Cough				
Sputum				

Stools # Daily _____ **Greasy, Yes/NO Color:** _____

Compression vest frequency: _____

Compression vest settings:

Intervals	Duration	Speed
1		
2		
3		

Pep Device frequency: _____

Additional Notes:

_____

_____

_____

_____

_____

Date: _____

Dispensed Medications:

Creon _____mg # with meals _____ # with snacks_____

	Dosage	Time
Breakfast		
Snack		
Lunch		
Snack		
Dinner		
Snack		

*Creon should always be given with a meal or snack, if it has been more than two hours since the last dosage. Do not administer generic brands of Creon.

Medication	Dosage	Times
Prevacid/Gas		
Albuterol		
Pulmozyme		
Saline		
Multi-Vitamin		
Specialty Vitamin		
Oral Antibiotic		
Inhale Antibiotic		
Nasal Spray		
Miralax		

Daily Activity

Special dietary needs:

_____
_____
_____
_____

Exercise: _____

	None	Light	Medium	Severe
Cough				
Sputum				

Stools # Daily _____ **Greasy, Yes/NO Color:** _____

Compression vest frequency: _____

Compression vest settings:

Intervals	Duration	Speed
1		
2		
3		

Pep Device frequency: _____

Additional Notes:

_____
_____
_____
_____
_____

Date: _____

Dispensed Medications:

Creon _____mg # with meals _____ # with snacks_____

	Dosage	Time
Breakfast		
Snack		
Lunch		
Snack		
Dinner		
Snack		

*Creon should always be given with a meal or snack, if it has been more than two hours since the last dosage. Do not administer generic brands of Creon.

Medication	Dosage	Times
Prevacid/Gas		
Albuterol		
Pulmozyme		
Saline		
Multi-Vitamin		
Specialty Vitamin		
Oral Antibiotic		
Inhale Antibiotic		
Nasal Spray		
Miralax		

Daily Activity

Special dietary needs:
_____
_____
_____
_____

Exercise: _____

	None	Light	Medium	Severe
Cough				
Sputum				

Stools # Daily _____ **Greasy, Yes/NO Color:** _____

Compression vest frequency: _____

Compression vest settings:

Intervals	Duration	Speed
1		
2		
3		

Pep Device frequency: _____

Additional Notes:
_____
_____
_____
_____
_____

Also by Heidi Wildes Mitchell

Novels:

Footsteps in the Attic

Footsteps in the Basement

Footsteps in the Galley

The Psychic Detective and the Editor

The Lady of Lake Ossahatchee

Short Stories:

The Elevator

Rattlesnake

Log Books:

Swimmer's Competition Log

www.ingramcontent.com/pod-product-compliance
Lightning Source LLC
Chambersburg PA
CBHW071532220526
45469CB00003B/748